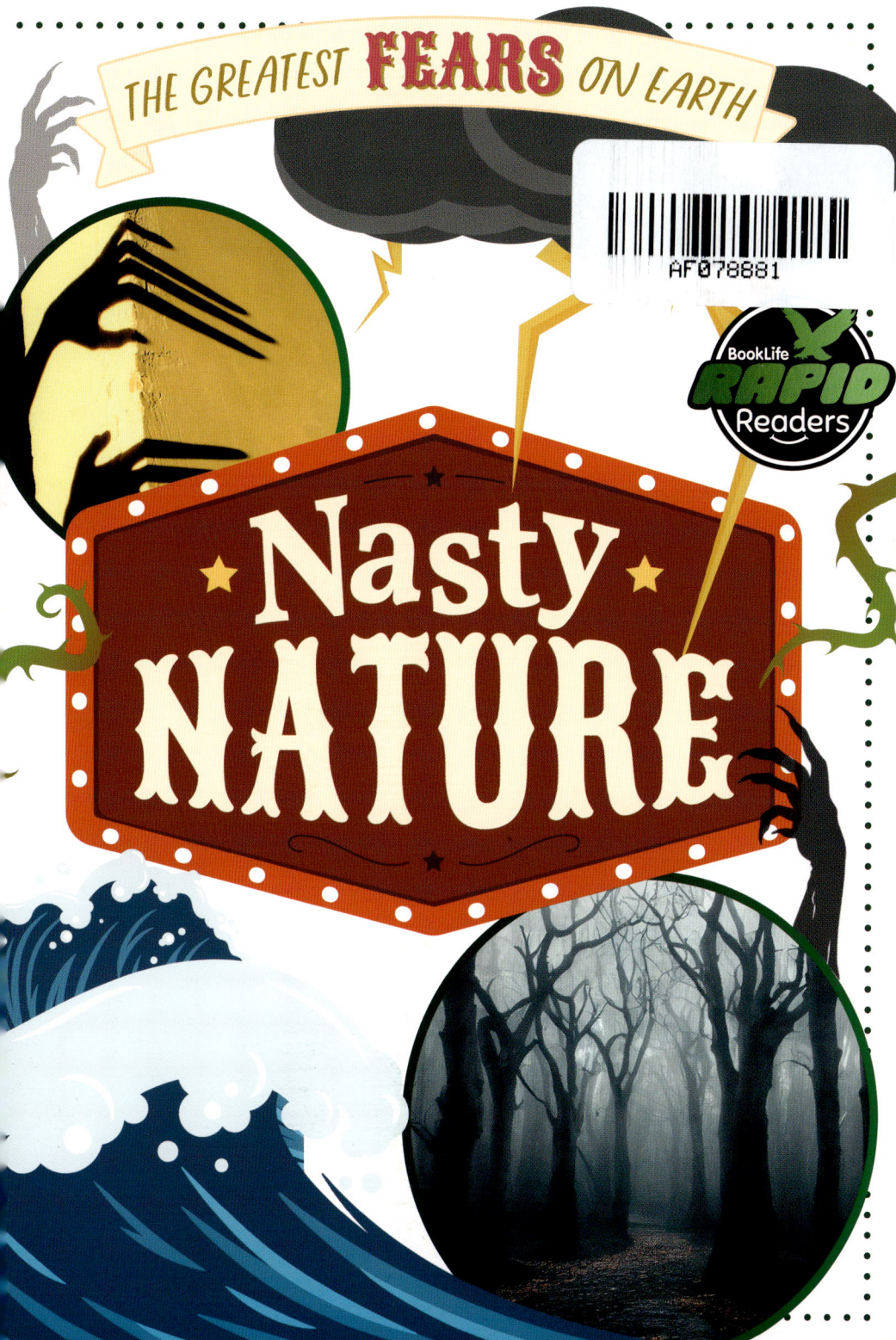

BookLife PUBLISHING

©2023
BookLife Publishing Ltd.
King's Lynn, Norfolk
PE30 4LS, UK

All rights reserved.
Printed in China.

A catalogue record for this book is available from the British Library.

ISBN: 978-1-80505-029-2

Written by:
John Wood
Adapted by:
Noah Leatherland
Edited by:
Kirsty Holmes
Designed by:
Jasmine Pointer

FSC
www.fsc.org
MIX
Paper from responsible sources
FSC® C113515

All facts, statistics, web addresses and URLs in this book were verified as valid and accurate at time of writing. No responsibility for any changes to external websites or references can be accepted by either the author or publisher.

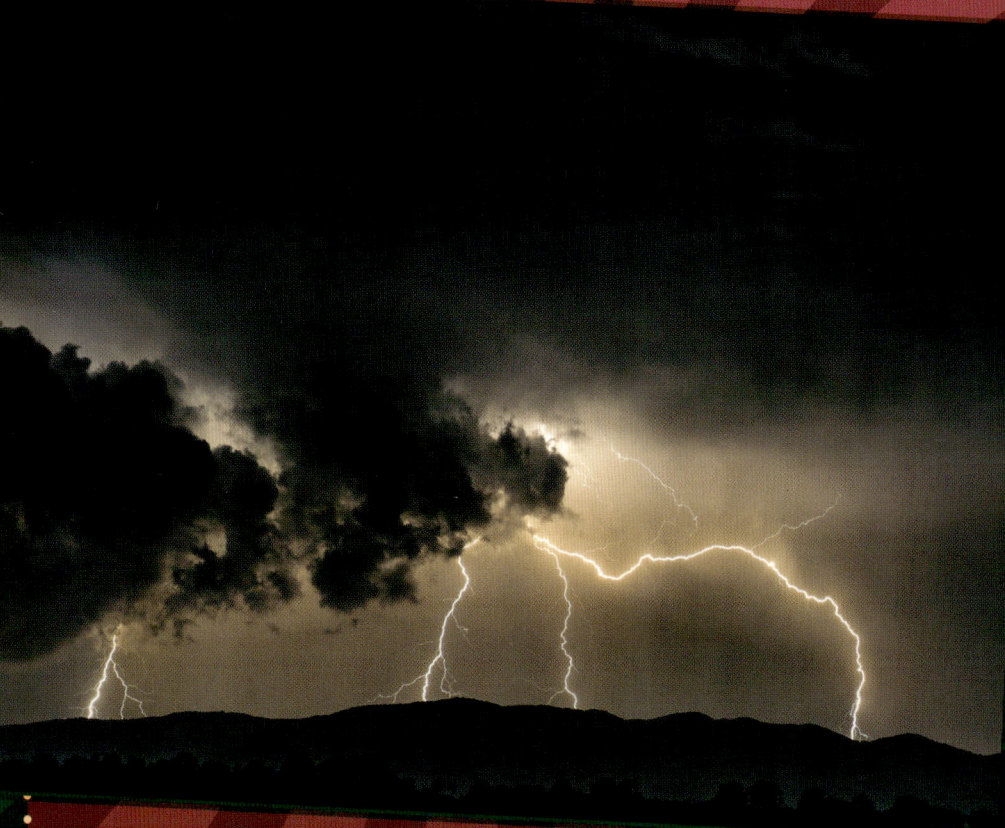

Photo Credits

Images are courtesy of Shutterstock.com. With thanks to Getty Images, Thinkstock Photo and iStockphoto.
RECURRING – pikepicture, kantimar kongjaidee, MagicMary. COVER – Sochillplanets, dhtgip, Kozlovskiy Andrey, Toma Stepunina, Macrovector, Denys Koltovskyi, OP38Studio, KLUSER. 4–5 – sicegame, Tom Wang, Mad Dog. 6–7 – andrejs polivanovs, Aastels, Inspiring. 8–9 – nutsiam, unjiko, EsHanPhot, Anton-Burakov, Dzm1try, Ammak. 10–11 – Darlene Wagner Butler, Pongsak14, dgultig, Butterfly Hunter. 12–13 – Macrovector, gie23, Vasin Lee. 14–15 – Diwas Designs, Yannick Morelli, M-SUR, Ludovic Farine, Mima40. 16–17 – altafulla, Lukasz Pawel Szczepanski, AJR_photo, Vectorpic, PodiumStore. 18–19 – Pimonpim T, Toma Stepunina, SusIO. 20–21 – Photo Spirit, Denis Andricic, Platoo Studio. 22–23 – natrot, r.kathesi, Elena Chevalier, Amado Designs. 24–25 – Vadim Sadovski, nami chwang, mapman, PrintablesPlazza, Tomacco. 26–27 – farzand01, maxbelchenko, VikiVector. 28–29 – superjoseph, Nicolas-SB.

CONTENTS

Words that look like this are explained in the glossary on page 31.

Page 4 Welcome to the Show!
Page 6 Worrying Waves
Page 8 Plant Peril
Page 10 Holes of Horror
Page 12 Thunder Fear
Page 14 Our Guest Star
Page 16 Light Fright
Page 18 Shadow Shudder
Page 20 The Science of Fear
Page 22 Dingy Darkness
Page 24 Big and Scary
Page 26 Scary Sickness
Page 28 Creeping in the Deep
Page 30 Curtain Close
Page 31 Glossary
Page 32 Index

WELCOME TO THE SHOW!

"COME ONE, COME ALL! COME AND SEE SOME OF THE GREATEST FEARS KNOWN TO HUMANITY!"

We have all felt fear in our lives. But do you have a phobia? A phobia is a strong fear of something, such as spiders or flying.

People have phobias of all sorts of things. Some people have phobias of things where there is no real danger.

The things you will see in our show were found all over the world. These are all real fears. Are you ready to find out what scares people the most?

Who knows, maybe you will leave the show with a brand-new phobia of your own?

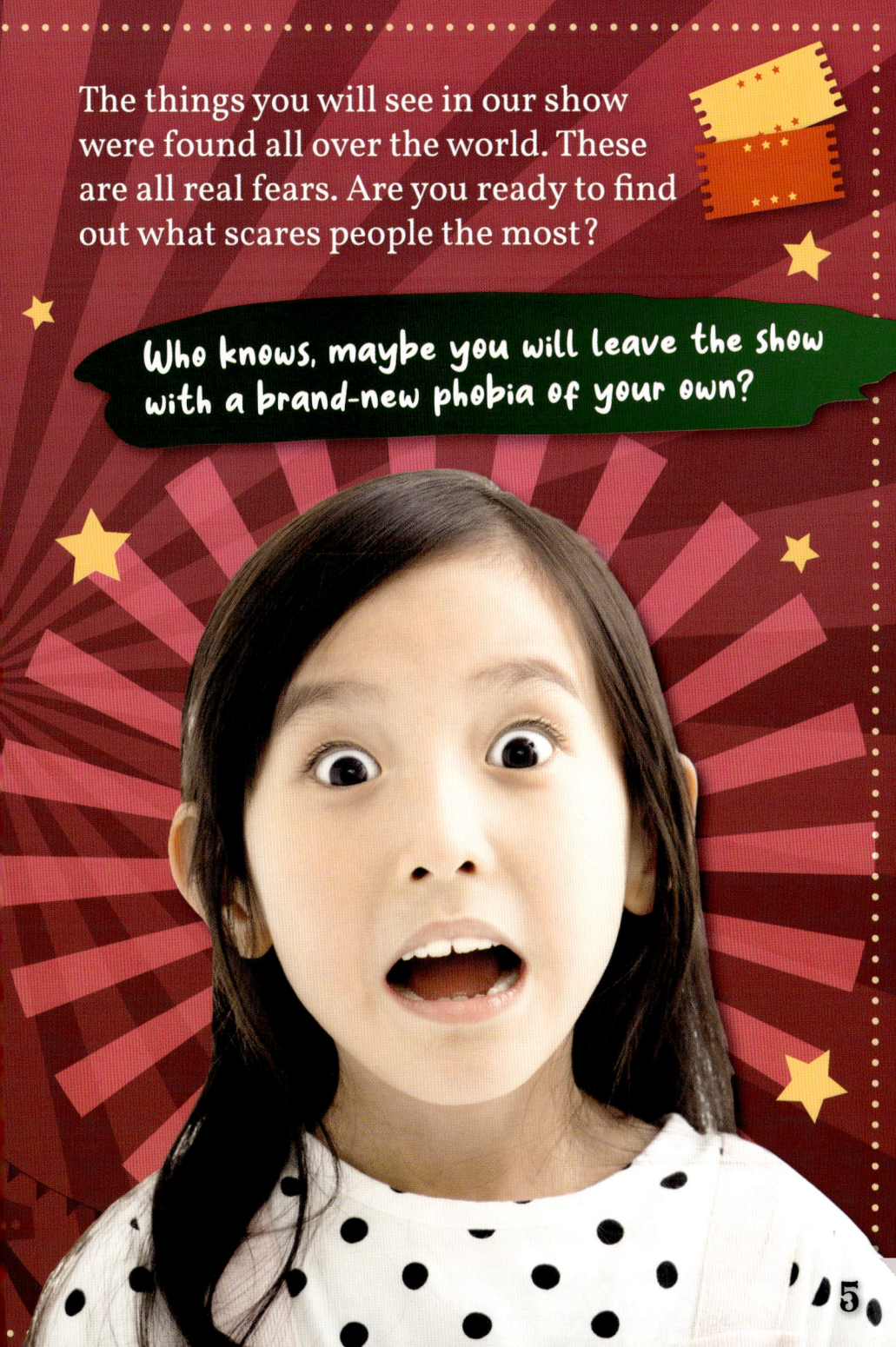

WORRYING WAVES

Waves are some of the most powerful forces in nature. It is no wonder that some people are afraid of them.

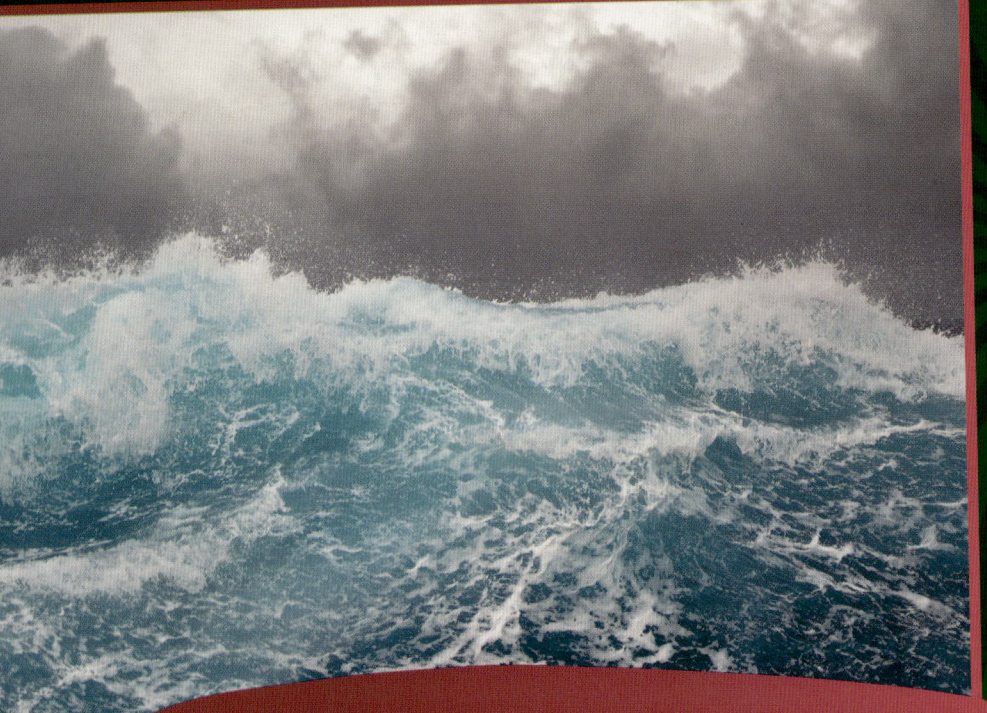

These things might slow down, but they never, ever stop. Over time, they can eat away at rocks and cliffs. They have shaped how the world looks for millions of years.

In a storm, waves can cause a lot of damage. They can tip over boats and can break things built on the coast.

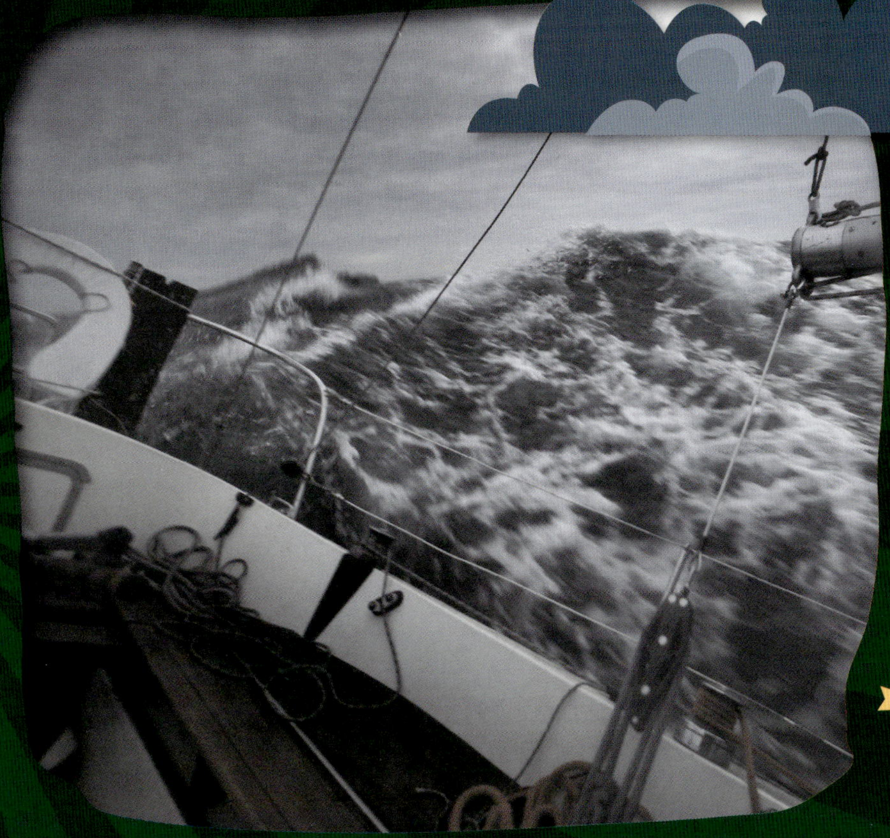

Waves of around 20 metres high have been recorded. That is about as high as four giraffes standing on top of each other. Can you imagine a wall of water like that rushing at you?

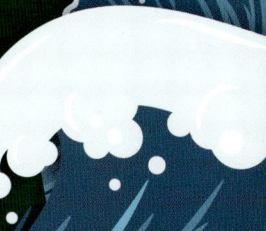

PLANT PERIL

Ever so slowly, they grow and grow. Across the ground, up the walls and deep into the dirt. They move slower than you can see, creeping towards the sun.

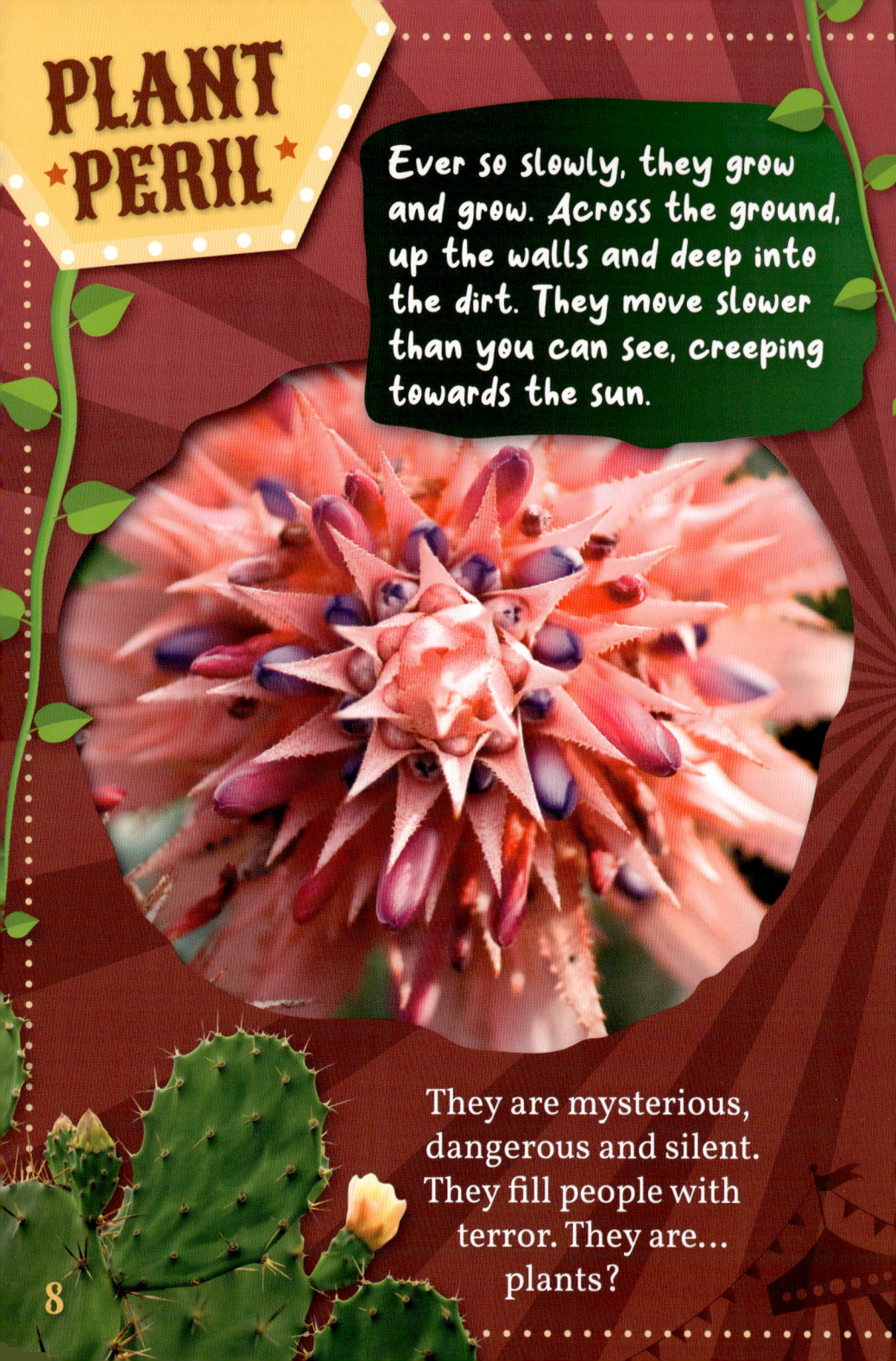

They are mysterious, dangerous and silent. They fill people with terror. They are... plants?

They might
not chase us, but
plants can be very dangerous.
Some plants have traps that eat
animals alive. Other plants are filled
with poison that can kill you if you eat them.

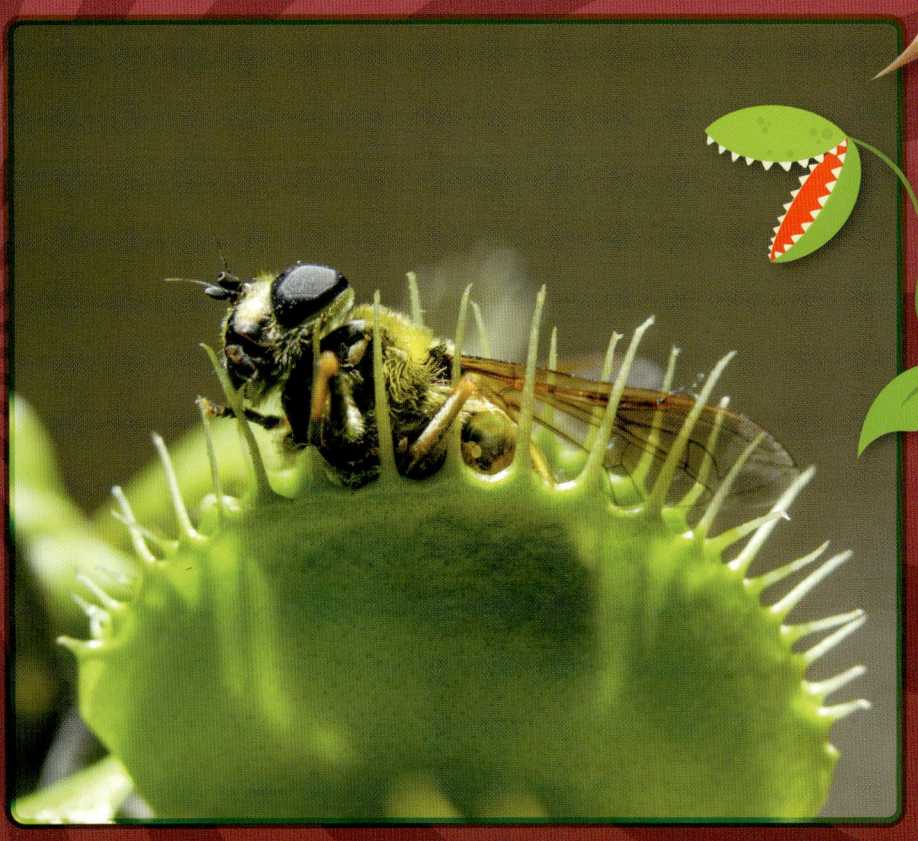

Some plants can hurt you and cause a lot of pain if they are touched. They might prick you with thorns or sting you with nettles.

HOLES OF HORROR

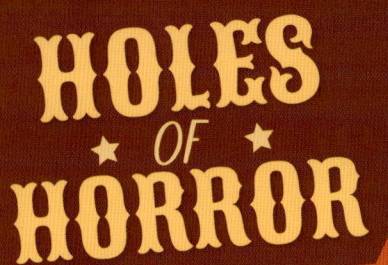

Do you feel that? On your hands? Hundreds of tiny holes in your skin!

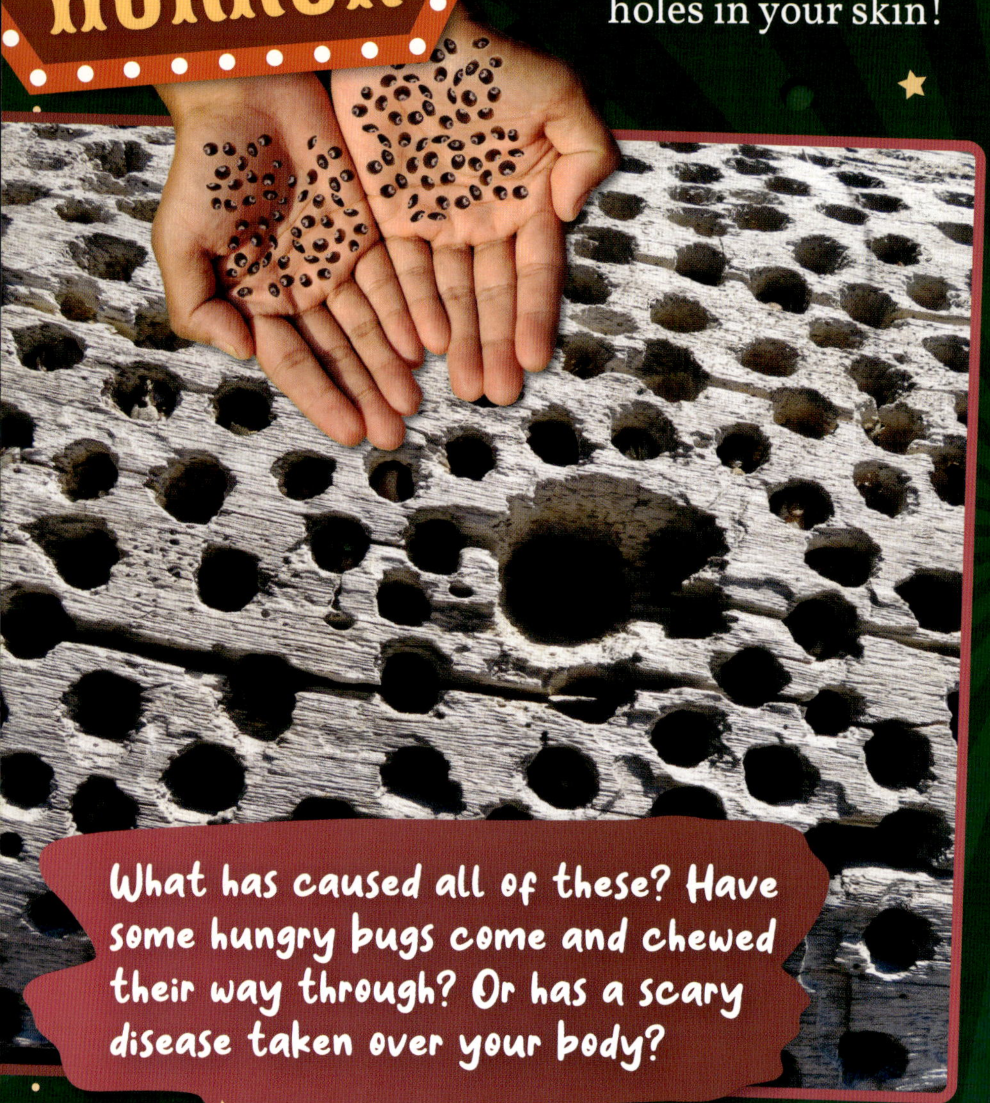

What has caused all of these? Have some hungry bugs come and chewed their way through? Or has a scary disease taken over your body?

The holes are so deep and dark you cannot see the bottom of them.

This is the fear of <u>clusters</u> of tiny holes. Though it is unlikely that your hands will suddenly be full of holes, you might come across these clusters in the wild.

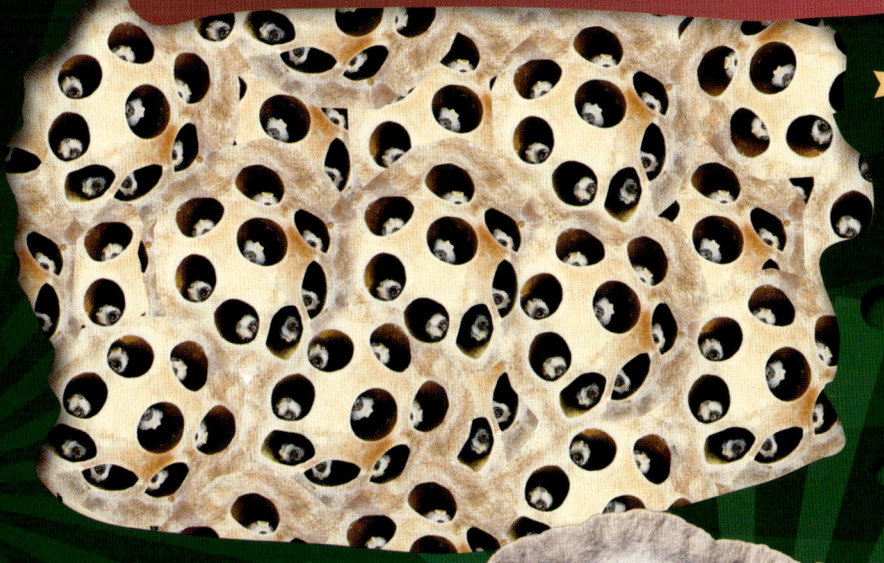

Some rocks naturally have lots of holes in them, and some plants have lots of holes that hold their seeds. People with this phobia cannot stand to look at them.

THUNDER FEAR

The black and grey clouds hang over your head and the rain starts to pour. You know it is going to happen, but when? You wait, and you wait, and you wait.

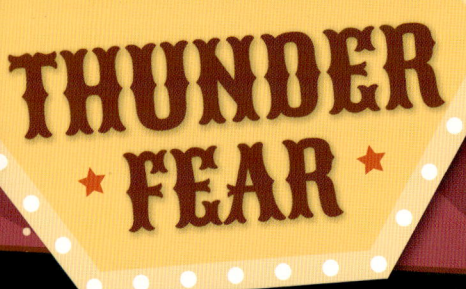

A flash of bright light in the dark. Then the sky booms with a loud clap of thunder. For some people, there is nothing scarier than thunder and lightning.

The fear of thunder and lightning is the third most **common** phobia amongst children in the US. Are you scared of thunder and lightning? Do they make you jump out of your skin?

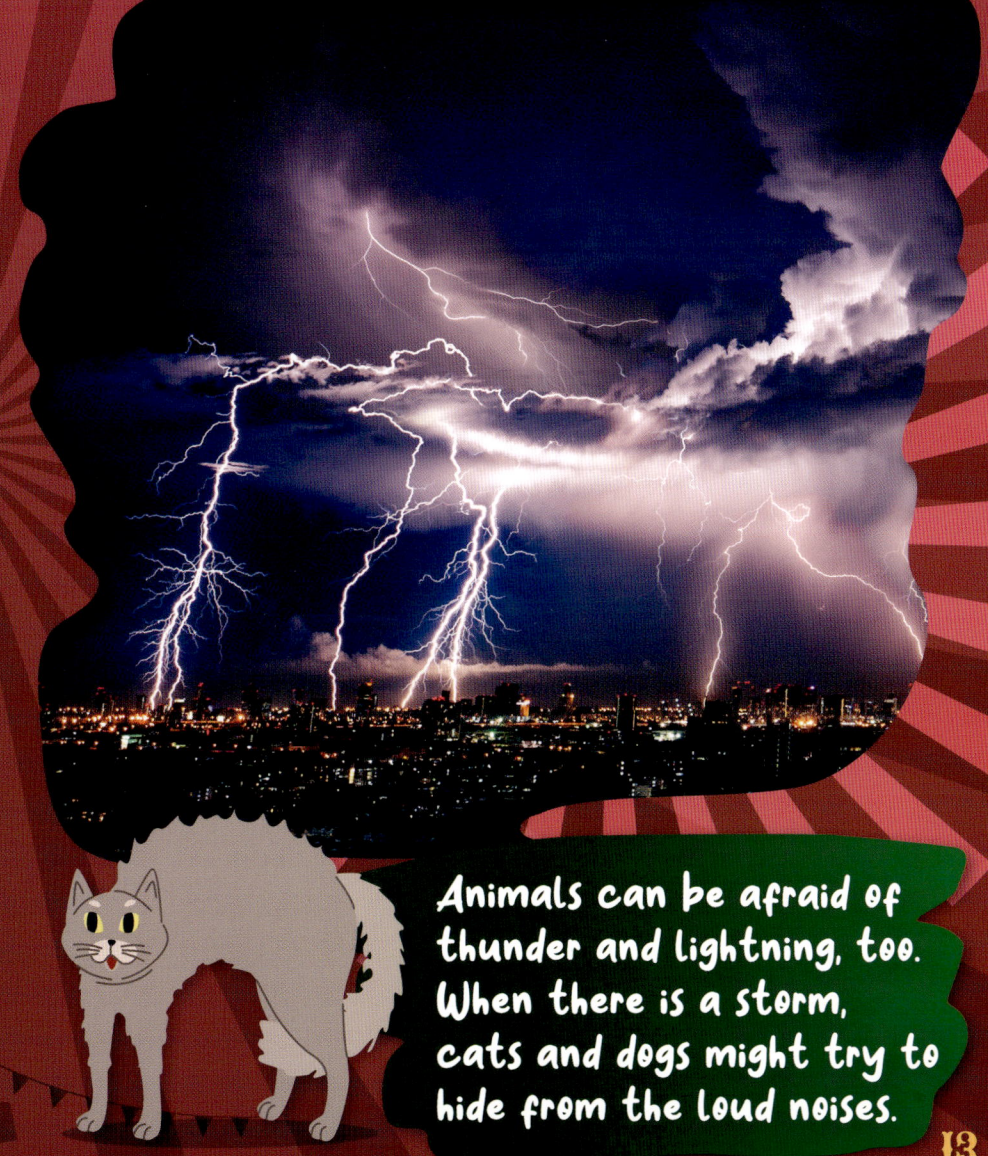

Animals can be afraid of thunder and lightning, too. When there is a storm, cats and dogs might try to hide from the loud noises.

OUR GUEST STAR

Augustus was the emperor of Rome over 2,000 years ago. Emperors were very important people. They ruled over all the countries that the Romans had taken control of.

Augustus was a very smart leader, but he could also be very mean. Sometimes, if someone he knew said or did something he did not like, he would have them sent away forever!

As well as being a <u>cruel</u> and powerful leader, Augustus had some phobias that terrified him. He was scared of lightning.

One day, Augustus was walking when someone in front of him was hit by lightning. Augustus thought that was a sign from the <u>gods</u>. He made sure a <u>temple</u> for the god of thunder, Jupiter, was built.

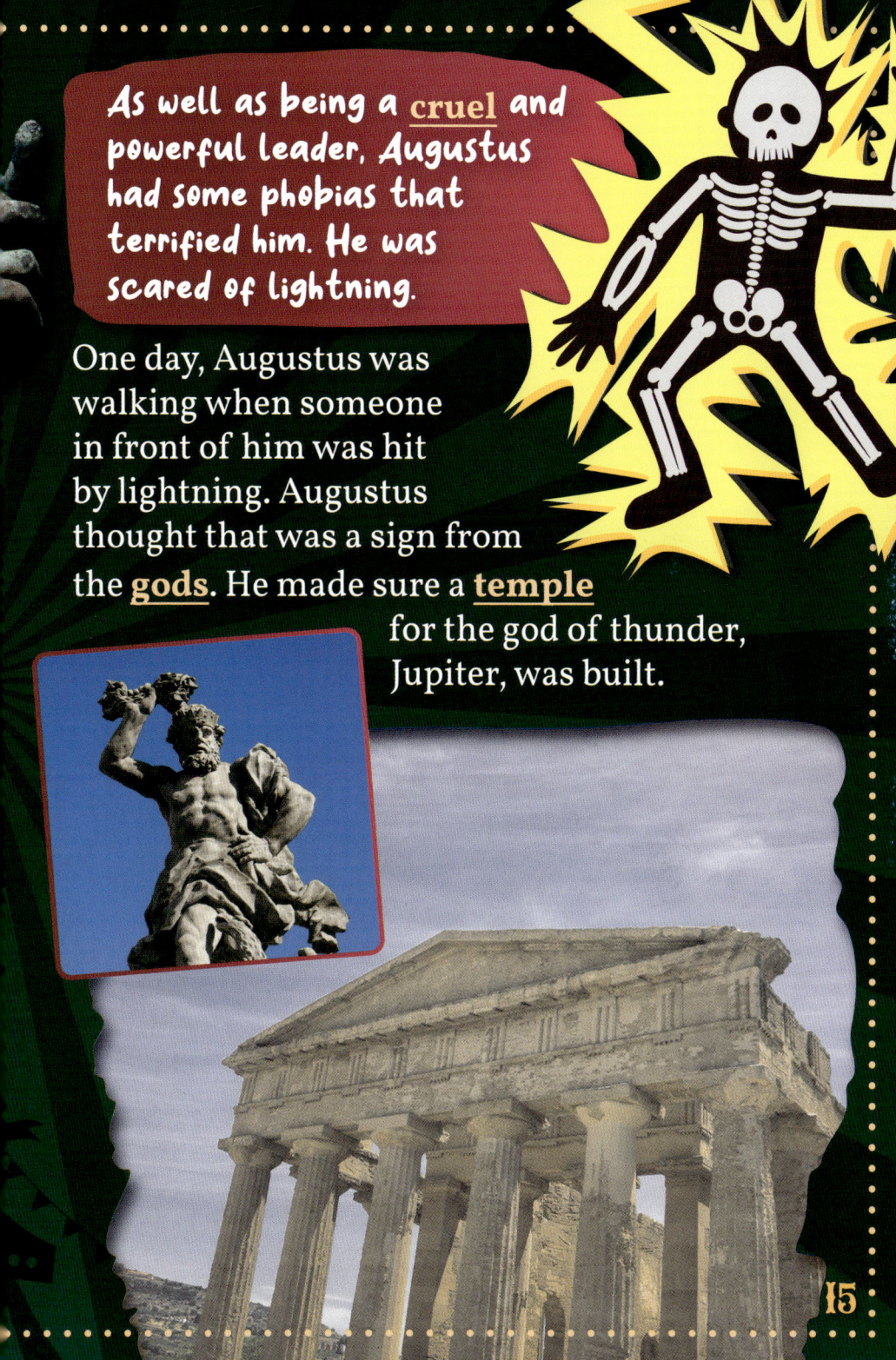

LIGHT FRIGHT

Plenty of people are afraid of the dark, but what about the opposite? Have you ever been scared of the light?

The Sun sits in the sky for hours. It is so far away, but it is so strong that it can still reach us and other planets. It covers our bodies, gets in our eyes and makes everything hot.

People with the fear of bright light worry about what sunshine might do to them. They are scared about getting sunburn or feeling unwell from the sun.

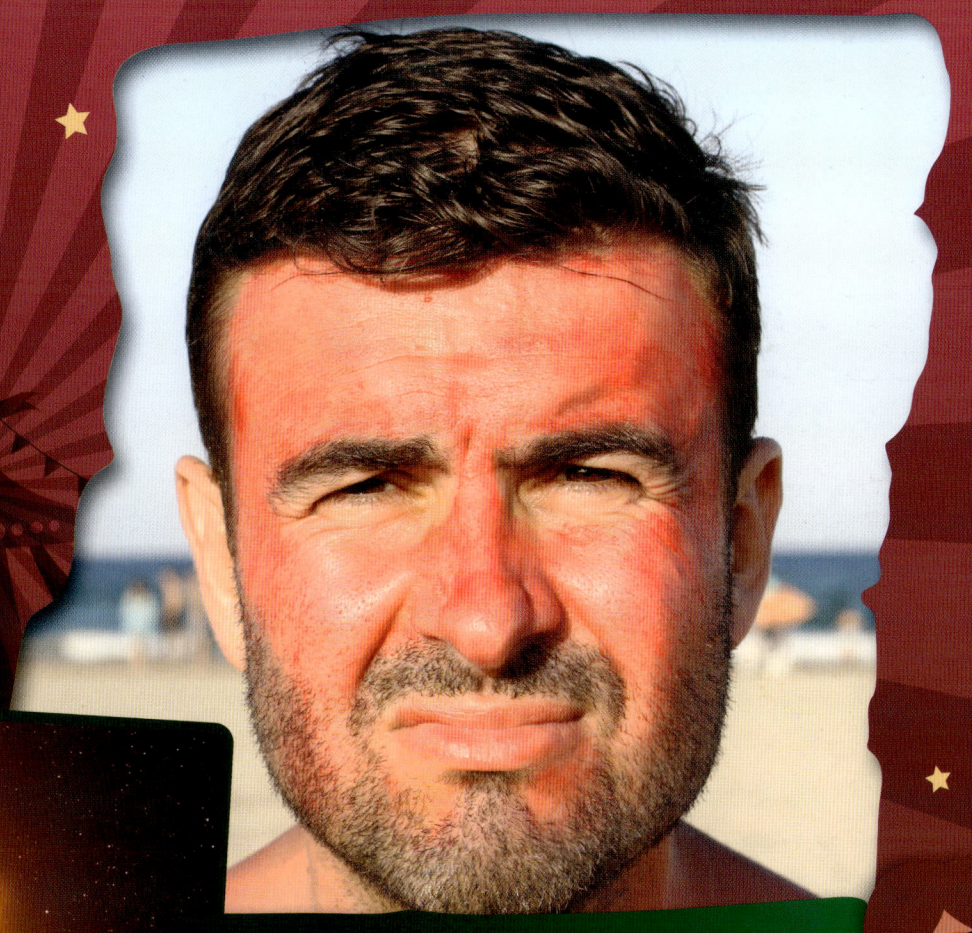

People with this phobia might cover themselves up as much as they can during the day. Or they might only go outside when it is dark.

SHADOW SHUDDER

Everyone and everything has one of these. They follow you everywhere you go. Sometimes they are small, sometimes they are huge. They are dark and mysterious. Sometimes, it is hard to tell where they are coming from.

> They are our shadows. No matter what we do, they will always be there wherever we go.

For some people with a fear of shadows, it is the way that shadows stretch and make us look like creepy monsters that scares them. For others, it is the way they move across the walls and the floor.

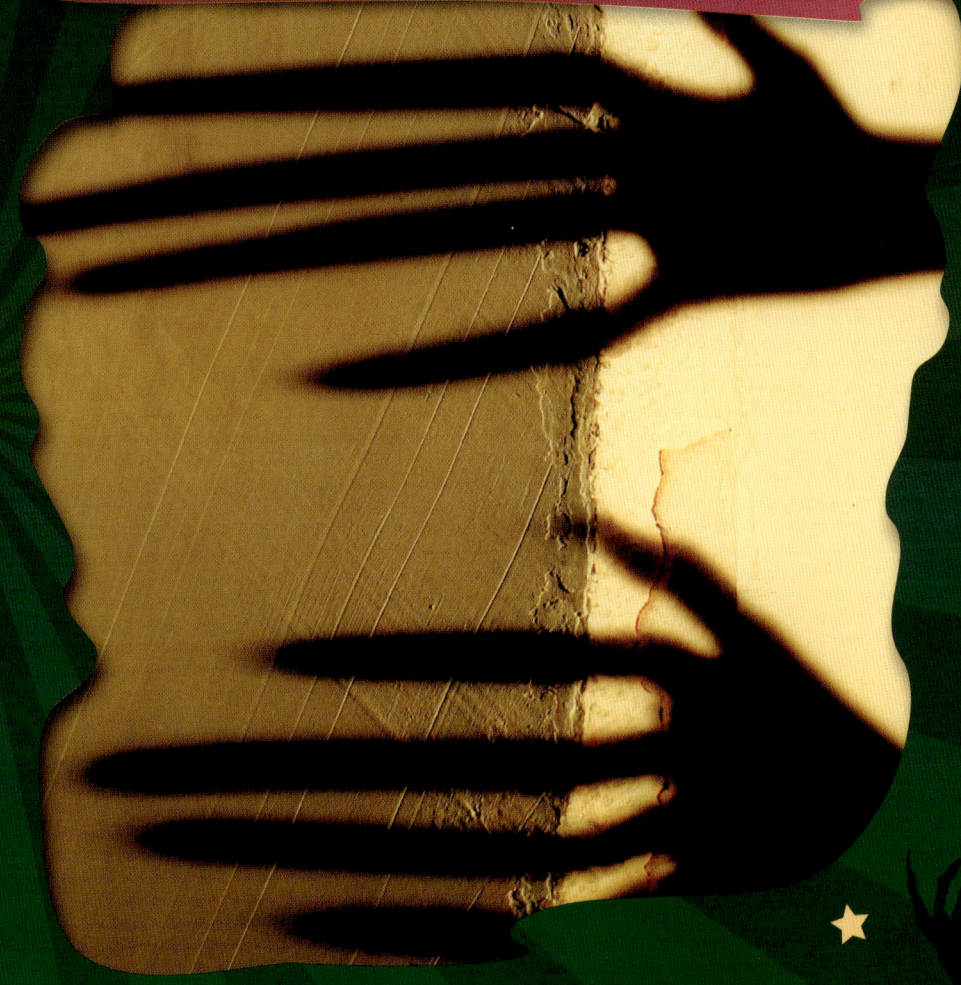

Next time you see your shadow, see how scary you can make it look.

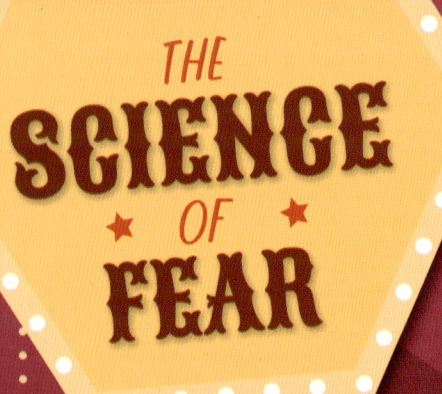

THE SCIENCE OF FEAR

Some scientists think phobias are caused by evolution. Evolution is how people and animals change over time.

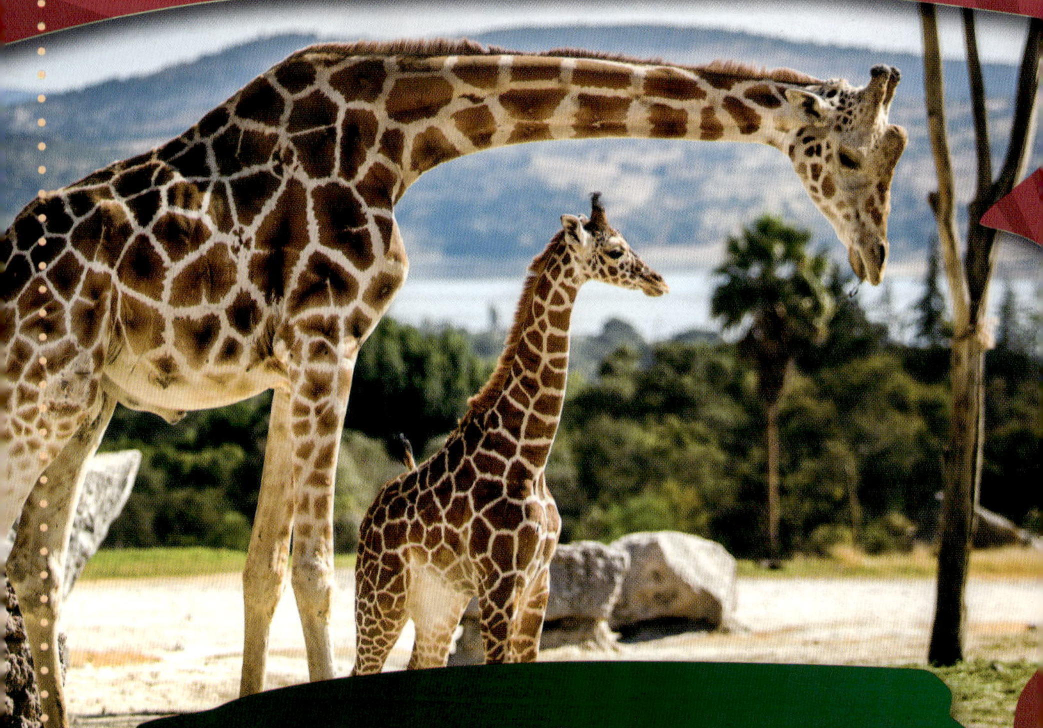

Children are often like their parents. For example, a giraffe with a long neck will have baby giraffes with long necks. A long neck helps them reach leaves high on trees and survive. The long-necked giraffes survive and, over time, the others die out.

Scientists think some phobias are passed down through evolution. Some of our phobias today might have been useful thousands of years ago.

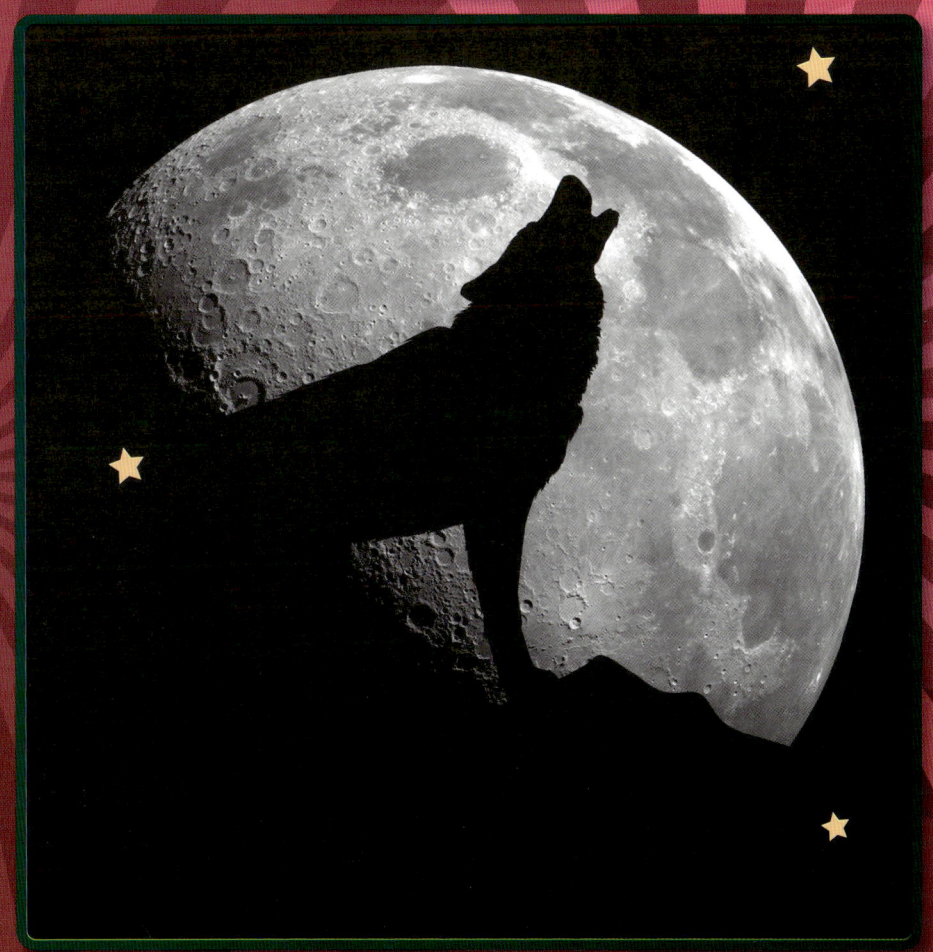

Being afraid of the dark might have helped the first humans when they were hunting in the wild. It is hard to see deadly animals in the dark, so being afraid of the dark helped them survive.

DINGY DARKNESS

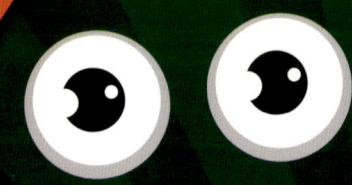

You cannot see a thing. The room is in total darkness. Your eyes dart around trying to see something, anything... but all you see is black.

In the dark, other things become clearer. You can hear the sound of your own breath. But... what was that? Is there something in the room with you? It is too dark to tell...

A lot of people have a fear of the dark. Most children are afraid of the dark when they are young. It is completely normal. Some adults have this phobia, too.

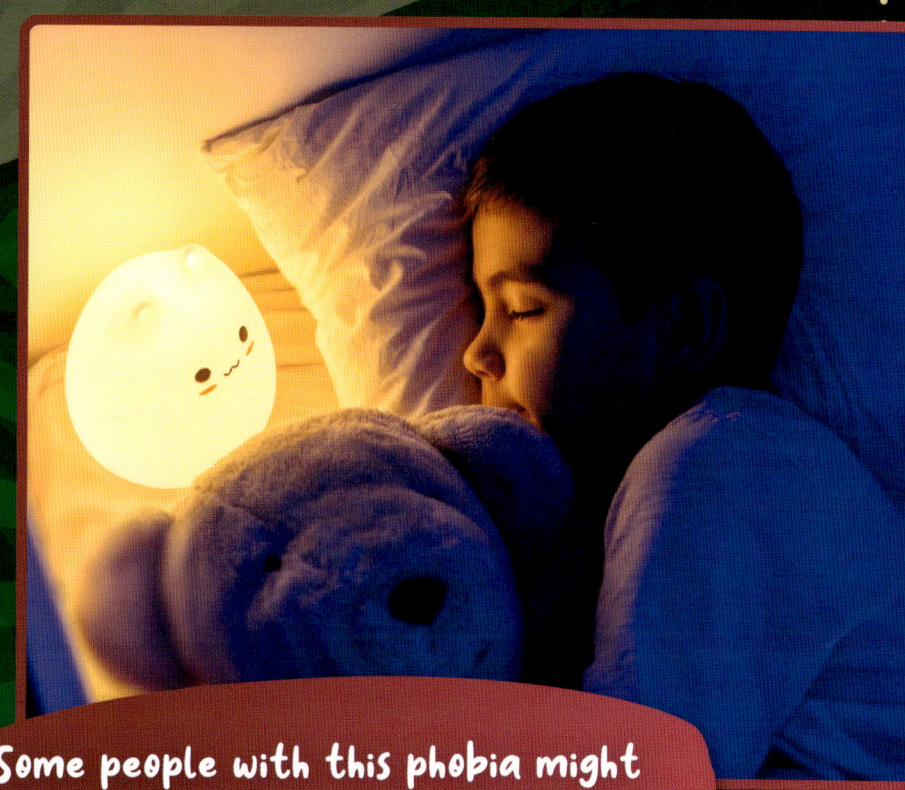

Some people with this phobia might struggle to sleep if it is too dark. They might need a nightlight to help them feel safe during the night.

BIG AND SCARY

Jupiter is bigger than all the other planets **combined**. There is a giant storm on Jupiter that is bigger than Earth. If Jupiter swapped places with the Moon, it would fill a huge amount of the sky.

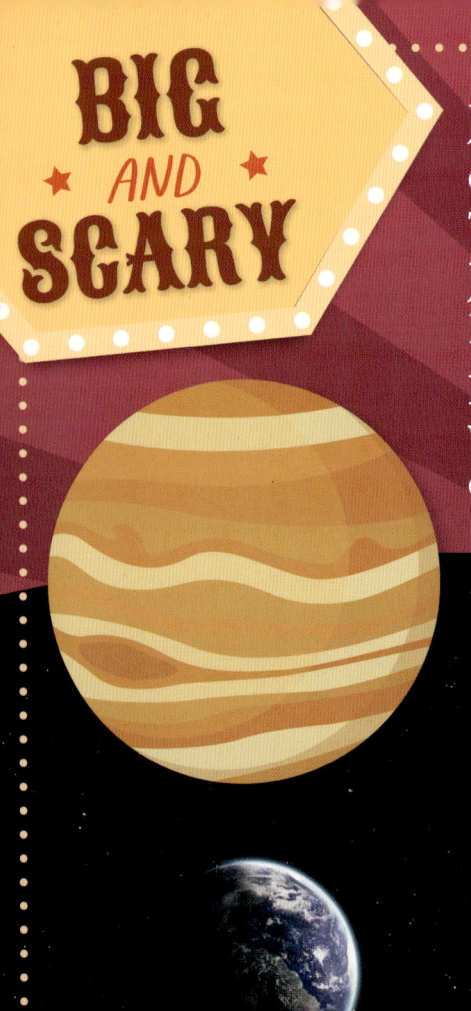

It would hang over you, bigger than anything you have ever seen. It would be too big to escape from.

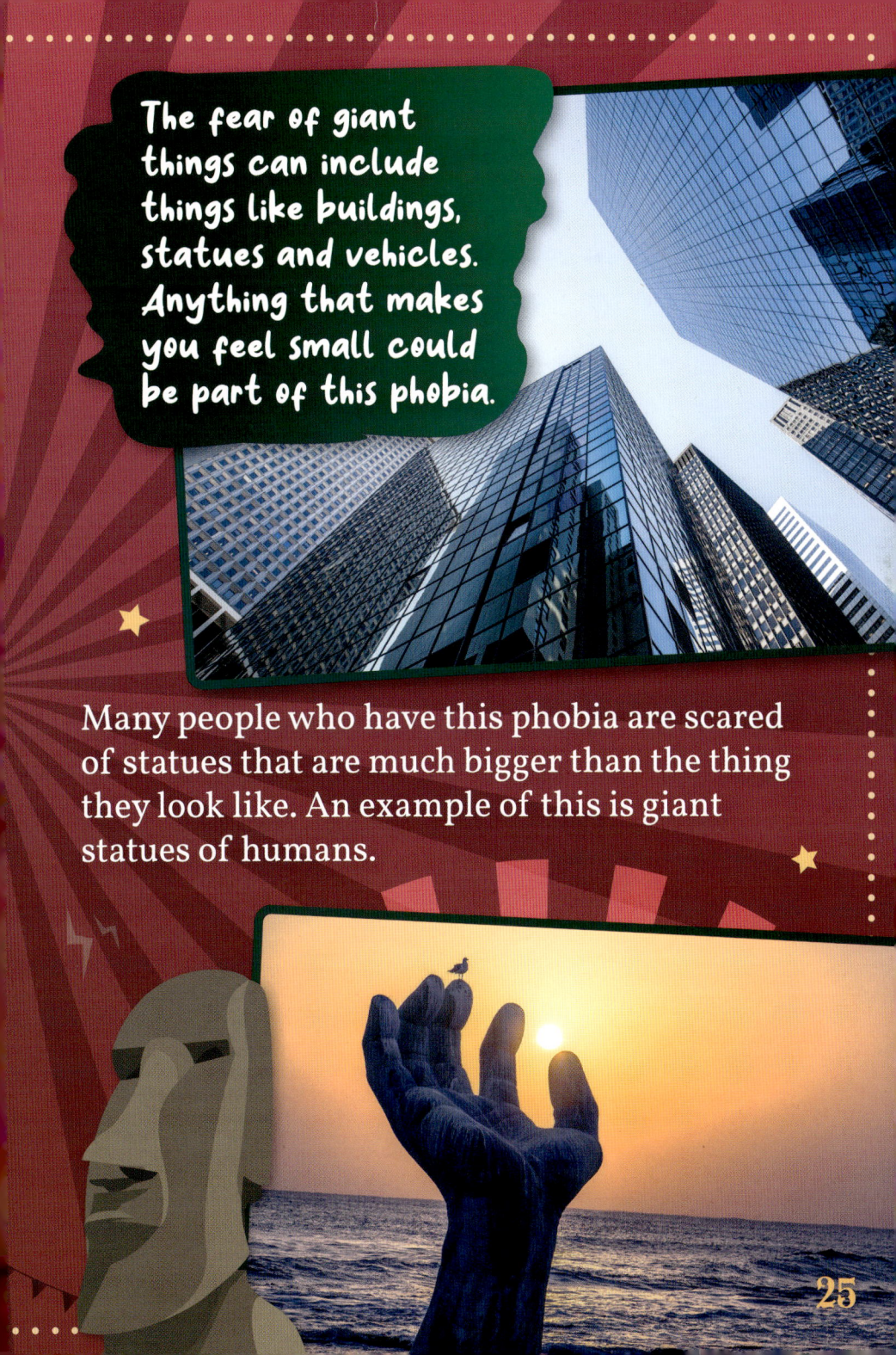

The fear of giant things can include things like buildings, statues and vehicles. Anything that makes you feel small could be part of this phobia.

Many people who have this phobia are scared of statues that are much bigger than the thing they look like. An example of this is giant statues of humans.

SCARY SICKNESS

How are you feeling today? Are you well? Or is there something making you feel unwell?

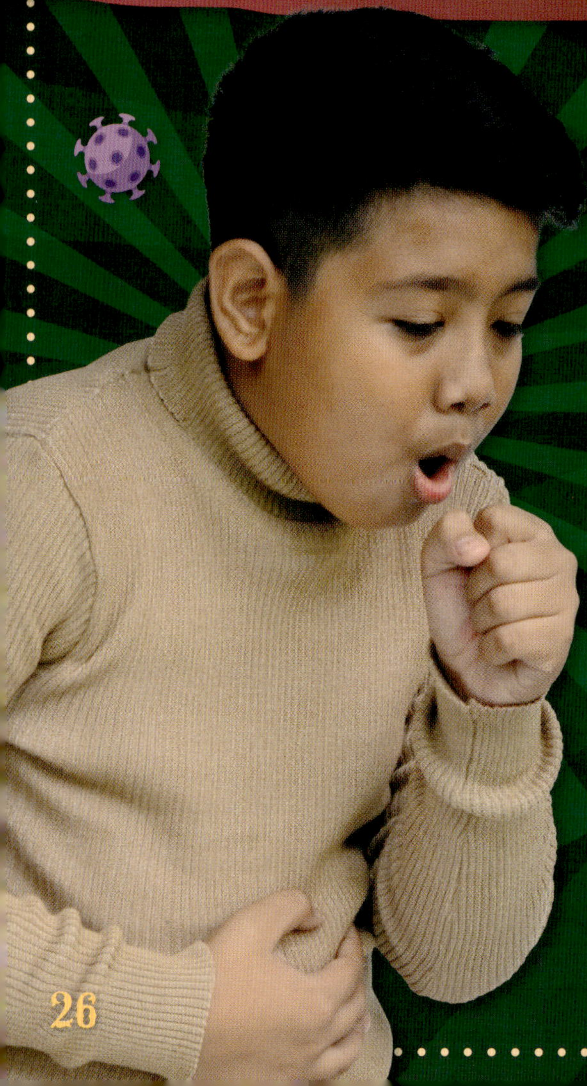

When you have a cough, do you ever worry that it is something more? Maybe there is something much more serious happening in your body that you do not know about.

The fear of an illness might make someone act extra carefully. They might clean more, cover themselves up or might not even leave the house.

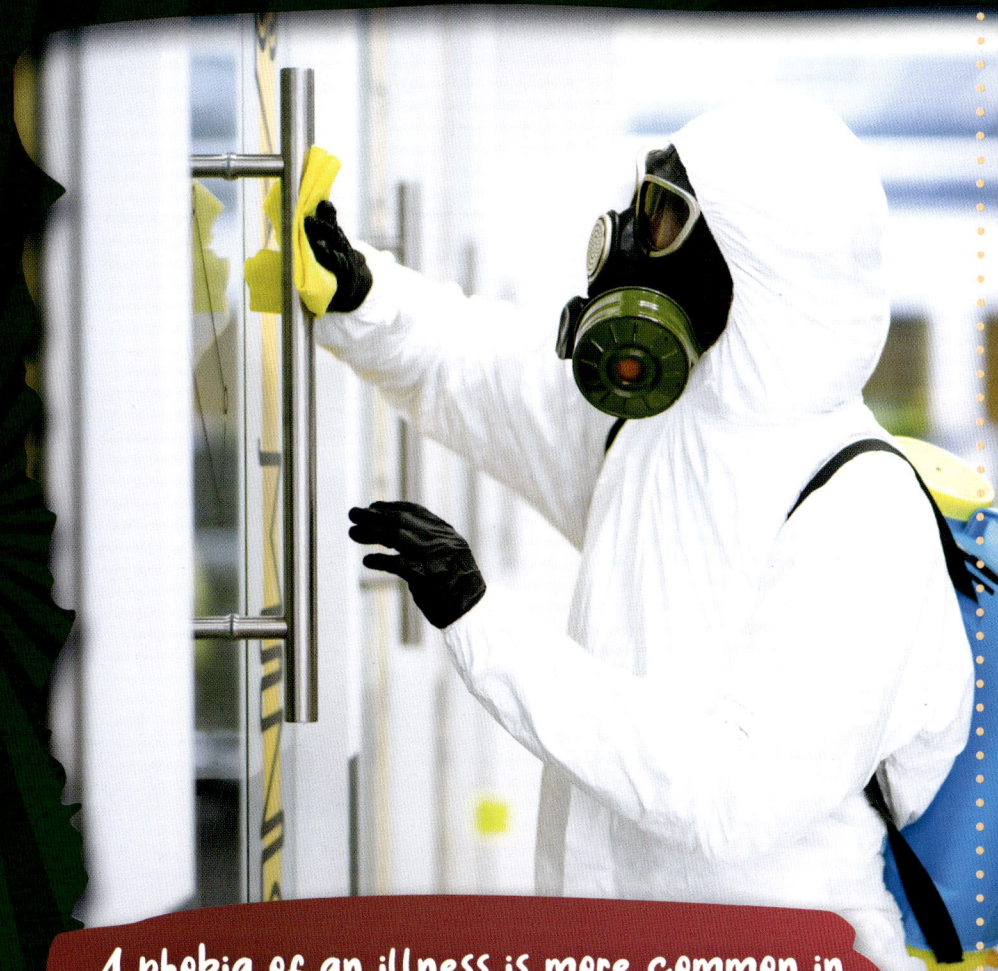

A phobia of an illness is more common in doctors and people who study diseases because they think about illnesses a lot. Sometimes just watching TV shows about illnesses can cause this phobia.

CREEPING *IN THE* DEEP

The oceans are very deep. The deeper you go, the darker it gets. There are still a lot of the Earth's oceans that have not been explored yet. Who knows what is waiting down there?

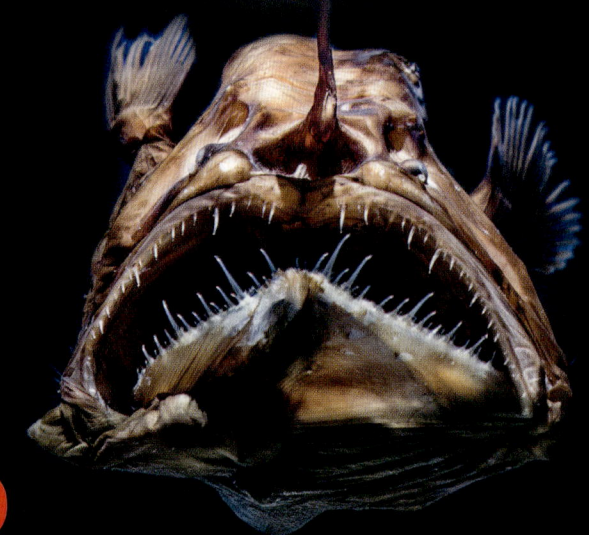

Creatures with sharp teeth? Long tentacles? Slippery scales? Whatever is down there, it would be impossible to see them. Fancy going for a swim?

Light usually does not travel more than 200 metres below the surface. In fact, everything below 1,000 metres deep is completely dark.

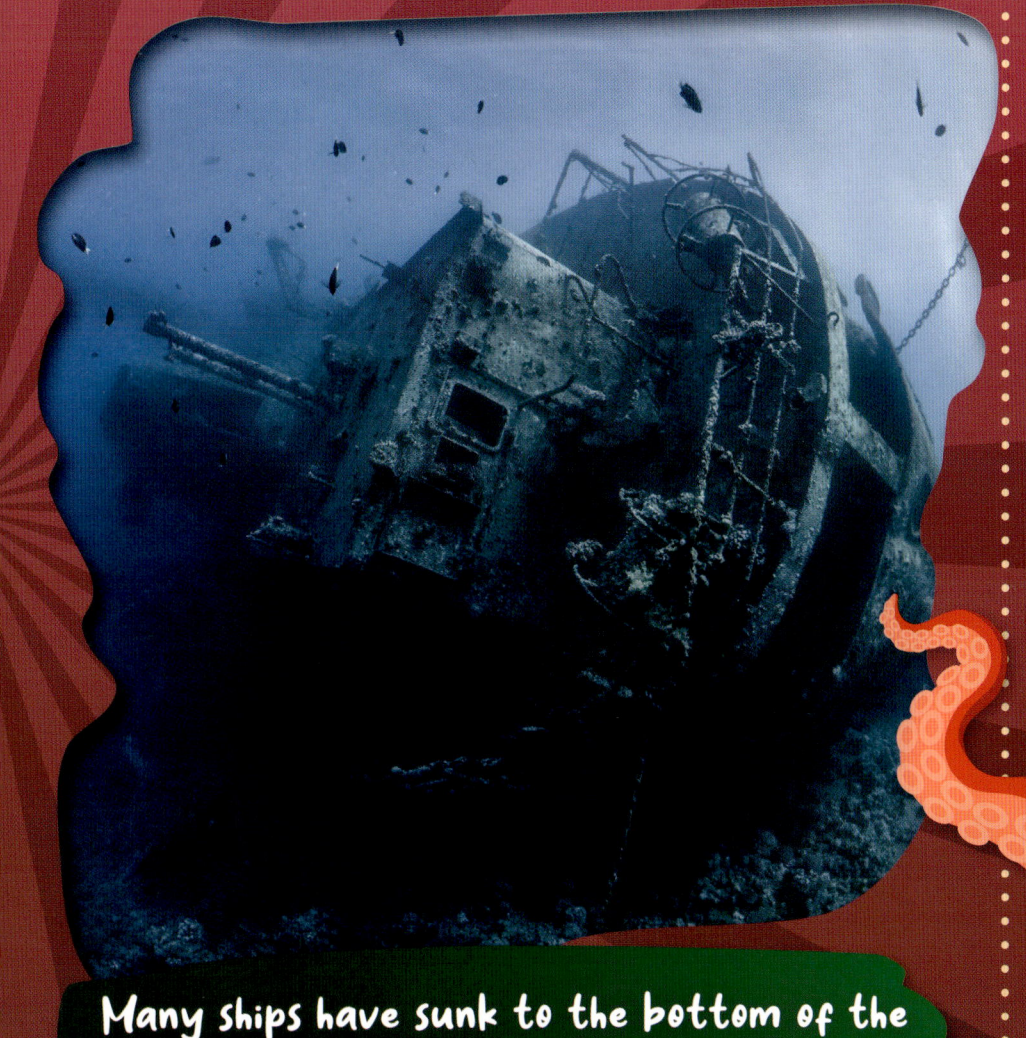

Many ships have sunk to the bottom of the ocean. But because the sea is so deep, they have never been found again. What would you find if you went down there?

CURTAIN CLOSE

AND THAT IS OUR SHOW! WE HOPE YOU HAVE ENJOYED YOUR JOURNEY THROUGH THE PHOBIAS. NOT EVERYONE IS ABLE TO GET TO THE END.

We have seen a lot of phobias, but there are plenty more things to fear out in the world. Did you find something new to be afraid of? We hope you are brave enough to come again...

GLOSSARY

clusters   groups of things close together

combined   joined together

common   often found

cruel   mean, unkind

gods   beings that are believed to be more powerful than humans

temple   a religious building made to give honour to important figures in a religion

INDEX

animals	9, 13, 20–21	lightning	12–13, 15
Augustus	14–15	oceans	28–29
darkness	12, 16, 21–23	planets	16, 24
illnesses	27	plants	8–9, 11

AN INTRODUCTION TO BOOKLIFE RAPID READERS...

Packed full of gripping topics and twisted tales, BookLife Rapid Readers are perfect for older children looking to propel their reading up to top speed. With three levels based on our planet's fastest animals, children will be able to find the perfect point from which to accelerate their reading journey. From the spooky to the silly, these roaring reads will turn every child at every reading level into a prolific page-turner!

CHEETAH
The fastest animals on land, cheetahs will be taking their first strides as they race to top speed.
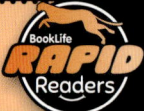

MARLIN
The fastest animals under water, marlins will be blasting through their journey.

FALCON
The fastest animals in the air, falcons will be flying at top speed as they tear through the skies.